How Yoga Really Works

by Jax Pax

Contact Details

To join my email list and keep up to date with my writing, please email me at:

counterintuitivethought@gmail.com

"For anyone interested in Yoga, Jax sifts through the complex maze of information about this ancient practice. He uses his knowledge on the subject, offering a well-researched, science based dialogue, alongside his personal experience as a practitioner. It is practical and can easily be used as a quick reference book for teachers, as they navigate questions from students. The author's careful reasoned analysis validates yoga's extraordinary healing potential."

Christine
Internationally Certified Iyengar Yoga Teacher
Massage Practitioner/Bodyworker

"This is a fascinating read, which clearly, in simple terms explains the physiological benefits of yoga. It is entertaining and easy to comprehend. Thank you for bringing forward scientific explanations, using critically assessed evidence to explain the real benefits of yoga."

Paulette
Internationally Certified Iyengar Yoga Teacher

Note to reader: I have written this book from a science-journalism perspective and, at the back of the book, I have included references to the claims to yoga's benefits mentioned throughout this book. While I have been practicing yoga for over a decade and I have more than half a decade of university level training in science and medical engineering, I am not a medical doctor. This information is intended for the reader's interest only and is not intended as medical advice. Consult a doctor before taking on any diets or exercises that may affect medical conditions.

Table of Contents

Introduction

Is yoga nothing but woo-woo? Hippy nonsense? And if it really works—how does it work—and what does it do exactly? In *How Yoga Really Works*, I will answer these questions from an observational or a scientific perspective as best I can and, I assure you, I'll get straight to the point so *you* can get straight to your practice! Let's get to it then.

What are the Benefits of Yoga?

"A rich man in a bad mood can feel destitute, and a poor man in a good mood rich beyond words." Anon.

So, what can yoga do for the practitioner? And what can it not? That depends on the style of yoga, the sequencing of the yoga session and various other factors.

Since there are now many different styles of yoga in existence, I will focus this discussion on the function of the most common styles of yoga such as Iyengar yoga and Hatha and I will exclude in particular Bikram yoga, Kundalini yoga and Ashtanga yoga. The primary reason for excluding Bikram, and Ashtanga yoga styles being that studies have found styles of yoga that emphasize cardiovascular fitness do so at the loss of other benefits such as relaxation and the lowering of the metabolism.

In the more stationary styles of yoga it has been found that yoga offers less benefit in terms of cardiovascular fitness.[i] But that's fine with me, considering the many other benefits that yoga does bring, and considering how simple it is to develop cardiovascular fitness through other activities. I, like most other people, do not go into yoga to improve my marathon time. We do it mostly for the benefits it has for the nervous system (and mind), for the skeletal muscles and joints, and for the endocrine system (hormonal).

In short, Yoga offers the following benefits. I will elaborate later in the book:

- Stress reduction
- Lowering metabolism
- Weight control (*despite* lowering metabolism)
- Craving control
- Mood regulation
- Treatment for depression
- Treatment for anxiety
- Increased flexibility
- Increased strength

- Increased bodily awareness

- Increased testosterone

- Benefits for childhood development

- Benefits for sleep

- Pain reduction

- Improved digestive health

- Healthy immune system

- Blood pressure regulation

- Slower ageing

- Treatment for food addiction

- Slower deterioration of the spinal discs and bones

- Yoga makes it easier to get out of bed

Why has yoga not yet received the credit it deserves in mainstream culture? Because you can't patent a natural therapy. Pharmaceutical medicine is much easier to make big business out of and therefore there is far more money that goes into scientific research for pharmaceutical medicine—and a hell of a lot more money that goes into marketing it too. Nevertheless, there is still adequate scientific evidence to support the claims for yoga's health benefits. This research has been going on for almost a century now. In addition to the scientific support, anyone who has committed to yoga practice with an effective teacher for a couple months can verify that yoga practice is worthwhile, to say the least.

How Yoga Works

To understand how yoga works we must first understand some basic principles from biological science. Fortunately, these are all easy to understand. I'll go through each relevant concept and we'll see how it all comes together.

The James-Lange Theory

To put it simply, the James-Lange Theory of emotion basically suggests that our brains are constantly monitoring our bodies and constructing emotions based on the nature of our physiological state. It turns out that this is at least partly true. While there may be more to the story—in that emotion is partly determined by cognition, awareness and perception also—nevertheless it is true that our bodily state does play a part in the construction of emotions.[ii] A big part.

There are studies showing that when people sit upright it enhances positive emotion.[iii] It has been found also that muscle-tone, i.e.—how tight your muscles are—affects anxiety levels. Yoga involves bodily gestures that exude confidence and openness such as the warrior asanas and open-armed asanas and it also leaves you with better posture throughout the day. All this contributes to a sense of freedom and resilience.

Homeostasis

> *To wing your course along the middle air;*
> *If low, the surges wet your flagging*
> *plumes;*
> *If high, the sun the melting wax consumes*
> —Daedalus to Icarus

Homeostasis means literally, *similar-state*. The body must maintain an equilibrium in order to function optimally. Body temperature, fluid balance, blood sugar levels, and many other factors need to be maintained at near optimal levels so as to avoid dysfunction and toxicity. As the body works to maintain a healthy balance chemically and physiologically this is called maintaining homeostasis.

However, the body cannot simply hold these factors statically at the optimal levels. Instead, it must maintain equilibrium by moving back and forth around a baseline. When individuals are unhealthy this function may be more chaotic or misaligned.

If we want to understand how yoga works, the concept of homeostasis is important in many ways, but most evidently, in regard to the nervous system. Put simply, if the nervous system is very turbulent, with energy swinging up very high and down very low, the individual will experience heavy mood swings.

Extreme moods not only tend to lead to painful experiences but also tend to coincide with distorted perceptions, and a tendency to seek drama or to see drama where there isn't any. Let's call it, *adrenalizing*.

So, all things considered it's often best to maintain a relaxed physiology and yoga provides an excellently effective way of doing that.

Breathing

Breathing techniques used in yoga really can affect the nervous system and can even enhance a person's decision-making capacity.[iv] [v]

Whenever you inhale, the sympathetic nervous system is activated slightly, creating a slight increase in heart rate. Exhaling does just the opposite: turning on the parasympathetic nervous system and activating your vagus nerve slows the heart as you exhale. This is why many breathing techniques practiced in yoga are built around extending exhalations. The breathing technique in which one gradually makes the out breath longer works by progressively slowing the heart and thus aiding relaxation.

Not all breathing techniques used in yoga are for creating calm however.

The Spine

"A striking aspect of the pain system is how readily it can be modulated by other factors. The strength of a pain signal, for example, can depend on what other sensory information is funneled to the spine at the same time. This, it turns out, is why it feels great to have a massage when you have sore muscles. Chronic, throbbing pain can be inhibited by certain types of sharp, brief sensory stimulation." — Robert Sapolsky, neuroendocrinologist [vi]

In yoga, great emphasis is placed on the spine. It is said that the spine is like the trunk of a tree. Without the trunk, the tree has no support, no strength, no conduit for the supply of nutrients (or in the case of the spine—nerve signals).

It has been observed that when the spine is compressed anxiety tends to be high and energy is low. In contrast, when the spine is erected and 'extended' there is more a sense of radiance and positivity.

It makes sense from a physiological standpoint that this would be the case. If the spine is compressed, as it is after four hours at the office desk for example, then the function of the thoracic organs will be compromised. An erect posture alleviates pressure on the organs and gives them space to function. It may be worth noting that it is well known that marathon running, which compresses the spine, can have a negative effect on mental health despite the runner's high that is experienced on running days.

In addition to the benefits coming from improved posture, yoga stretches and strengthens the muscles and other tissues around the abdominal and thoracic regions, thus allowing the spine, the rib cage, and the shoulders to open up, providing significantly more space for the organs to function without being inhibited by tight muscles. The lungs are then able to breathe more easily, and in turn the heart is able to relax a little more. The abdominal organs are given more space too, and the resulting improvement in function is easily felt by an experienced practitioner as she leaves her office desk and releases through a yoga workout.

A well-functioning spine supports the nervous system by supporting the organs that are linked with it. The heart, lungs and digestive system have a very significant effect on the nervous system and therefore affect our sense of well-being and freedom.

But there is an additional factor regarding posture that affects the psychological state also. Remember the James-Lange theory mentioned earlier? The observation that the brain monitors the body to determine the emotional state? Having an erect posture leads to greater confidence, relaxation and well-being by that effect also.

Not only does yoga develop the core support muscles that help maintain good posture throughout the day, but also, during the yoga session there are many postures (a.k.a. asanas) that exude superb confidence, openness and even humor. The warrior poses and salutations are examples of postures that instill such positivity.

Keeping the spine strongly supported, relaxed, and erect through yoga training leads to increased mental clarity, relaxation, and positivity.

If you are skeptical about the ability of yoga to have such significant effects on the nervous system try hanging from a pull-ups bar with your core muscles relaxed such that your body weight is pulling your spine into an extension as you breathe deeply through the diaphragm for ten breaths. If you go for a brief walk after the exercise you will likely notice an increase in mental clarity and overall positivity. Or better yet, try an 8-week beginner's course!

For another experiment, try doing a full hour-long workout that is focused on extension asanas. These asanas involve activating muscles around the spine that we don't make enough use of in modern life. The muscle activation involved is similar to pushing the spine into an extension, as if you are reaching up to bite something. You will find that after doing a long workout full of extension asanas you may not be able to sleep much that night. You will lie in bed feeling very alert and energetic. This is why the sequencing of a yoga session is usually designed in a balanced way. However, a class focused on extensions could be used if the situation calls for it. Maybe you want to be particularly alert for your day job, then a morning routine focused on extensions may be an effective alternative to a mug of coffee.

Heart Rate Variability

Increased *heart rate variability*, a measure of the variation in time between each heartbeat, has been found to be associated with increased emotional resilience and reduced anxiety and stress levels.[vii]

A well-sequenced yoga workout develops heart rate variability partly through breath training and partly through training the heart via movement between inversion postures and extension postures.[viii, ix, x, xi]

Inversion postures lower the heart rate while extension postures raise the heart rate. So, moving back and forth between the two throughout a yoga session effectively develops heart rate variability.

Another benefit that comes with moving between different postures—i.e. inversion to extension, or lying to standing—is that it becomes much easier to get out of bed in the morning. Getting up out of bed requires quite a change in the heart rate and this is more difficult if the heart has not developed fitness in that regard. Yoga sessions, in a sense, are great practice for getting out of bed.

Internal Locus of Control

Locus of control refers to the degree to which one believes that they, as opposed to external forces, have control over their lives. A person with an internal locus of control is one who believes that their perceptions have a lot to do with their own mindset and physiological state and that they can control outcomes in life, to some extent, by their own actions and attitudes.

Mastery in yoga leads to an increased awareness of how the physiological state affects perceptions of daily events and this then leads toward a more internal locus of control. The great thing about this is that you realize that sometimes you can fix—or at least reduce—a lot of problems by looking after your physical health and by practicing an effective mindset rather than needing to make the external changes that are often much more difficult to achieve. If your job seems like hell and you've been getting by on coffee and chocolate to boost your mood every day, switching to a healthier lifestyle with plenty of yoga and healthy food to calm the nerves and improve blood sugar regulation may lead to a very significant improvement in well-being, relaxation and enjoyment.

GABA

Studies have found yoga increases levels of the inhibitory neurotransmitter *Gamma Aminobutyric Acid* (abbreviated GABA).[xii] [xiii] GABA is a neurotransmitter that slows the firing of neurons, making them less excitable and thus leading to a reduction in anxiety. If information gets to the amygdala[1] faster it will be less accurate, so this slowing of the brain signals is actually helpful for accurate perception.[xiv] The calming effects of increasing GABA are thought to be another factor that contributes to yoga's effectiveness as a method for anxiety reduction.

A 2007 study demonstrated that the brains of yoga practitioners showed an average GABA rise of 27 percent, while the control group (those not

[1] The amygdala is a brain region associated with emotional processes and motivation.

practicing yoga) showed no rise whatsoever.[xv] The yoga practitioners who were most experienced and practiced most frequently showed particularly significant rises in GABA. One study participant was measured to have a GABA rise of 47 percent and one participant had an increase of 80 percent while practicing five sessions per week.

Another study compared the effect of taking up Iyengar yoga to regular walking. The participants had no previous yoga experience and practiced Iyengar yoga as they learnt it from scratch for three months. The results showed an average GABA rise of 13 percent which was significantly better than the walkers.[xvi]

Balancing Asanas and Improved Concentration

Practicing balancing asanas—such as handstands or asanas involving standing on one leg—is a great way to improve concentration and still the mind. Balancing requires full-body awareness and consumes much, if not all, of one's attention. The result is not only that there is peace of mind during the asana but also there tends to be an enduring ability to concentrate effectively throughout the day after performing balancing asanas.

Blood Pressure

During times of acute stress, the body has adapted what scientists call the *stress response* as a way of dealing with situations where it is fight-or-flight-to-save-your-neck. Such situations require rapid mobilization of energy as your muscles are going to be working like crazy.

Glucose and the simplest forms of proteins and fats come pouring out of your fat cells, liver and muscles, in aid of whichever muscles are saving your ass. Once all that glucose has been mobilized it needs to be delivered to those muscles as quickly as possible. That means heart rate, breathing rate, and blood pressure need to increase in order to transport the nutrients at optimal speed.[xvii]

The trouble is, we humans have the potential for rumination over past events and the potential to anticipate future stresses that may or may not be going to occur. And so, while the stress response is very useful on the savannah as you are dodging to save your ass, in modern life it has become a potentially lethal health hazard in itself. While there is certainly some utility in worrying about potential future stresses, much of the time our daily stress is wasted energy. Rumination rarely solves problems. And worrying about the mortgage too heavily probably isn't aiding you in your financial management ability. Chronic stress is likely to create more problems than it solves in the domains of health, finances and relationships.

Yoga reduces blood pressure partly by reducing stress and partly in more direct ways.[xviii] [xix] [xx] [xxi] [xxii]

(see also: section—How the Shoulder Stand Works)

Weight Loss is Not About Will Power: Yoga Stops You Reaching for the Fridge

During chronic stress, glucocorticoids (basically the stress hormone) circulate the body. At these times when glucocorticoid levels are high it has been found, both in humans and in rats, that some individuals become *hyper*phagic under stress while others become *hypo*phagic under stress. *Hyper*-phagic means the individual is driven to eat more while *hypo*-phagic means the individual loses their appetite.

But increased appetite is not the only change that can result from raising glucocorticoids. Glucocorticoids stimulate appetite preferentially for foods that are starchy, fatty and high in sugar.

By reducing stress levels, yoga lowers the presence of glucocorticoids circulating throughout the body. The result is that you now have less to fight against. Your cravings change—you want junk food less and salad more. See, it's not a matter of will power or self-discipline—the cravings simply aren't there anymore. You no longer feel the need to be rescued by cake.

Changed cravings in combination with raised *whole*-body-awareness and suddenly the junk food doesn't seem so appealing. The cola might stimulate your tongue but it will put a weight on your heart. When you are stressed you feel as if you're exercising your freedom by eating tasty junk. But when you are relaxed, radiant, and lucid after a yoga workout, the sweet junk foods feel as if they are overly forceful, *pushing* your physiology to behave in a predictably reactive way rather than *allowing* the body to be responsive to the actual situation of the day.

Testosterone

"Life is not only stranger than we have imagined. It is stranger than we can imagine."
J.B.S Haldane, biologist

Looking at the research it can be confirmed that it is a myth that testosterone plummets with age.[xxiii] It turns out that the changes in testosterone levels depend on the individual. One thing can be confirmed however—in general, it is stress, not age, that leads to plummeting testosterone levels.[xxiv]

Another myth is that sexual behavior and violent behavior is directly correlated with testosterone levels. Actually, this too depends more on the character of the individual and even reducing an individual's testosterone to 10% of its normal level does not affect sexual behavior much.[xxv] [xxvi]

Since yoga is effective at reducing stress levels, it may assist at keeping testosterone at a healthy level and maintaining the bodily functions that follow that. One study found that testosterone levels rose, on average, 57% in men and in some individuals, testosterone doubled after a course of yoga.[xxvii]

A Russian study published in 2004 found the cobra asana could reduce the stress hormone cortisol by 11% on average, while testosterone rose by 16%. Men showed increases in testosterone that varied from 2% to 33%. But, as with many physiological benefits that have been found to come from yoga, the effect appeared to be much stronger in females than in males. The testosterone levels of the study's lone female continued to rise, eventually reaching 55%.[xxviii] The difference may have something to do with the fact that women produce much of their testosterone in their adrenal glands.

Another factor that is known to reduce testosterone is a vegetarian diet. So, yoga may be a good accompaniment to a vegetarian diet for its ability to buffer against this loss in testosterone.

It has been found too, that over-exercising decreases testosterone levels as the endorphins released during runners high inhibit testosterone release.[xxix] With this in mind, yoga may be preferable as a lighter alternative to more extreme forms of exercise (such as endurance sports and marathon running).

Digestive Health

"How intriguing, in this context, that the enteric nervous system—the complicated mesh of nerves that is present in our gastrointestinal tracts—so resembles old nerve net structures. This is one of the reasons why I suspect the enteric nervous system was really the "first" brain, not the "second", as it is popularly known." Antonio Damasio, neuroscientist xxx

It is a well-supported fact that lower stress means better digestive function. In the fight-or-flight scenario, digestion is put on pause while the *sympathetic nervous system* switches on to ensure that energy is going toward saving your neck rather than digesting that burger as you're dodging that grizzly bear.

In chronic stress, there is over-activation of the *sympathetic nervous system*. So, yoga's stress-reducing effects provide excellent support for the function and maintenance of the digestive system also.

If you are skeptical about yoga's ability to affect digestion, try this experiment: hold the shoulder stand for five minutes straight at the end of an hour-long yoga session and see if you need to go to the toilet soon after.

Immunity

"It seems pretty convincing that stress makes the common cold more common at least partially along the psychoneuroimmune route." *Robert Sapolsky, neuroendocrinologist* [xxxi]

Speaking from an evolutionary perspective, in the high-stress situation you would expect immunity to increase rather than decrease. And you'd be right, it does—at first.

Imagine you've just been bitten by a predator—now you're going to need raised immunity to fight off infection—and so evolution has endowed us with such a response to high stress situations, i.e. high-stress *initially* leads to raised immunity. But, keep that stress going over the long term and immunity plummets as shown in the graph below.[xxxii]

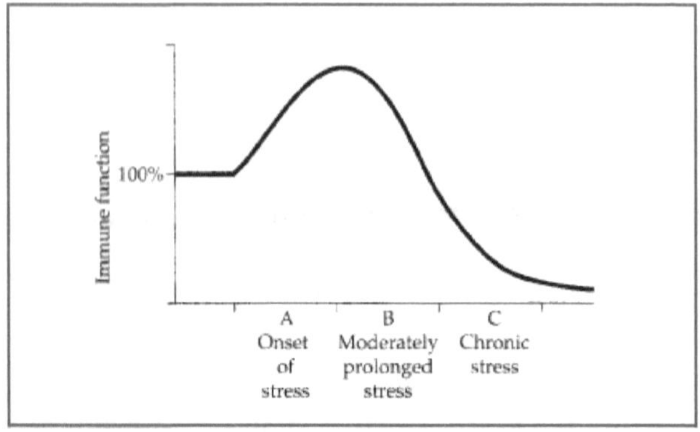

This graph is an illustration of how immune function increases at the onset of stress but decreases after prolonged stress.

And in modern life this is just the sort of situation we are so often thrust into. We don't just have today to worry about, we have the next thirty years to worry about. The mortgage, career success etc. And when your immune system is chronically activated, you've got yourself an autoimmune disease as the body begins to mistake parts of you for something invasive.[xxxiii]

Slowing Ageing

"Genes load the gun and the environment pulls the trigger." George Bray, Obesity Researcher

Scientists have found that while you are born with a particular set of genes, lifestyle factors can influence the way your genes express themselves. In 2009, the Nobel prize for biology went to Elizabeth Blackburn, Carol Greider and Jack Szostak for their research relating to telomeres. Telomeres are repeating segments of DNA found at the ends of your chromosomes and it turns out that the length of your telomeres is a good marker of your biological age. Shorter telomeres predict cognitive decline and other factors of ageing. And it so happens that one of the strongest predictors of telomere shortening is chronic stress.

Studies have found that relaxing meditation practices and Qigong (similar to Tai Chi) reduce stress and increase *telomerase*, the enzyme that replenishes telomeres.xxxiv While this is not quite yoga, the results are predictive of what could be expected from yoga as the researchers associate the telomerase increase with stress reduction.

Harvard trained physician, Dean Ornish, a long-time devotee of yoga known for his popular books on healthy living, conducted a study with 24 men ranging in age from fifty to eighty. The men practiced yoga for an hour a day, six days a week. Their telomerase levels and other physiological measures were assessed before the practice began and again at the conclusion of the three-month study. The study's results were admirable. Scientists found declines in blood pressure and cholesterol, and the participants reported less emotional distress and less disturbing thoughts. Remarkably, it was found that telomerase levels increased by 30%.xxxv

Studies by researchers Cliff Saron of the University of California and Quinn Conklin have similarly found positive effects for telomerase levels in correlation with meditation retreats.xxxvi

Aside from the relationship between meditation practices and telomerase, there have been studies showing that older people who've been practicing yoga for the long-term show less wear of vertebral discs, greater spine density, and improved balance.xxxvii These factors are very important considering that falls are one of the leading factors that lead to morbidity.

How the Shoulder Stand Works

The yoga researcher, Mel Robin, has proposed that the shoulder stand works largely by altering the regulation of blood pressure.[xxxviii] In the shoulder stand, the base of the front of the neck is at a bend and is being placed below the heart. This inverted body position allows gravity to aid venous flow right from the legs back down toward the heart. The right atrium of the heart is equipped with a sensor that gauges pressure.

At the beginning of the shoulder stand, as the blood pressure begins to rise in the right atrium, this raises alarm and initiates the parasympathetic nervous system's response to slow the heart to a gentler pulse. By this mechanism, the calming effects of the shoulder stand are realized. The body must have this adaptive response in order to prevent brain tissue from being damaged by excessively high blood pressure.

It is for this reason mainly that inversion asanas—the ones in which the head is below the heart—are effective at reducing anxiety. A large part of the benefit of yoga comes from cycling back and forth between inversions and standing postures or extensions multiple times during a session as this develops the hearts ability to change modes skillfully.

Development During Childhood

"Glucocorticoids atrophy neurons in the frontal cortex. By the time you are 14, stress has [potentially] made you unpopular because a well-functioning frontal cortex is linked with popularity." Robert Sapolsky, neuroendocrinologist xxxix

I attended pediatric mental hospitals and clinics where I discussed with the speech pathologists at length about what leads children into the facility. As you can guess, many of the children have hereditary mental health problems, and many have suffered a lot of abuse and domestic violence. What many people don't realize however, is that when children are subject to such extreme stressors during their developing years, the result can be a slowing or even a stunting of brain growth.

The first part of the brain to cease growing is the part that is least important for bear survival—the language centers.

As a result, many children who grow up under severe stress carry with them what speech pathologists call a *pragmatic language deficit*. This basically means they are stuck with the language skills of a younger person (perhaps a seven-year-old) permanently. Since language is so important for reasoning and comprehension and understanding other people's behavior, the pragmatic language deficit can potentially make it particularly difficult for these people to flourish in adult life and to have adult-like relationships.

While such cases are quite extreme, this reality does highlight the importance that a relaxed physiology has for a child's development. Not that children need to be floating in yoga bliss all their lives to grow and thrive, but it is important to keep in mind that high stress can be detrimental to a child's development and yoga may be an effective practice to include in a child's (and especially a teenager's) lifestyle if stress is becoming of concern.

How to Stick to Practice

"Exercise is stress-reducing so long as it is something you actually want to do." Robert Sapolsky, neuroendocrinologist [xl]

"We can easily forgive a man who is afraid of the dark. The real tragedy of life is when men are afraid of the light." Plato

An exercise plan of any nature can be challenging to stick with, but for many people, sticking with yoga practice is even more challenging than sticking to rigorous exercise. Why? Because when you contemplate yoga practice you aren't just confronting what at first seems like effortful work, you're also confronted by *The Unbearable Lightness of Being*. The more one lets go of physiological and mental stimulation, the more one develops a down-to-earth awareness of the present reality, but the flip-side to this can sometimes be that there is no longer the comfort of escaping into distractions.

This can sometimes result in long-abated dramas being re-presented as if the mind attempts to recreate the turbulent physiological conditions it had been used to, as in the situation of a drug-addict experiencing withdrawal symptoms. While yoga is mostly very enjoyable, there can be very uncomfortable periods while the body is recalibrating to the new level of neurophysiological arousal.

When you really think about it, the question—do I *feel* like practicing yoga today? —should be irrelevant. When you ask yourself that question you assess by drawing your awareness to the way you *feel* in that moment and if it is a negative, sluggish feeling you say—no, I don't *feel* like doing yoga today. If the decision as to whether or not you should do yoga is always decided upon in this way the answer will always be no. How can you *feel* like feeling elsewise? You cannot. It is contradictory. But you can *decide* you'd like to feel differently to your current state if you look to your values, to your best interests.

If, rather than motivation, it is time constraints or energy levels that are making it hard to practice, it's much better to do 10 minutes of yoga than none at all. In fact, you can get quite a lot of benefit just from 10 minutes a day. Even better, if you can manage multiple 10 minute sessions throughout the day in spare moments, that will be very effective at recalibrating the nervous system if practiced consistently. Remember the concept of homeostasis mentioned at the beginning of this book? Those large, over-shooting waves of high and low will calm down and smooth out a little if you allow frequent release of tension to become a regular habit. And for those readers who are confined to an office chair throughout the day—chair yoga is a real thing.

Here's a list of strategies to consider if sticking to practice is proving difficult:

- **Try shorter sessions.**

- **Don't wait for when you *feel* like doing it.** Just get the thing in motion.

- **Consider what is in your best interests.**

- **Think long term.**

- **Do it for yourself.** Do it for your own sense of freedom. Do it for your own clarity of perception.

- **Do it for your living partners.** The calming effects of yoga may make you a little better to live in a house with.

- **Don't do it for good looks.** Good looks are a demotivating goal because the more you focus on that the more you begin to notice the inevitable imperfections that you and every other human being have. And as those imperfections stand-out more and more, you begin to associate the negative feeling of focusing on your looks with exercise itself and eventually prefer a life of hedonistic escapism.

- **If you cannot spare the energy to workout, at least lie down on the mat.** Lying down on a yoga mat in savasana, has a different effect physically and mentally than lying on a mattress. And once you've been lying in savasana for a few minutes you might even be more inclined to do a few more movements.

- **Try chair yoga** or just do a few of the asanas you find to be most effective. Even just doing one asana may be very beneficial especially if you do it well.

- **Move the practice to a different time of day or night.** Different times of day have different effects. Practicing late in the day seems to make for a better sleep which then makes for a more relaxed morning and so that is the favorite time for many practitioners. Practicing in the morning can help make you feel radiant throughout the day but it can be very difficult to make the time in the morning.

- **Change the sequencing of the asanas.** (for something new)

- **Develop your skills.** Developing new skills can help to keep the yoga interesting and may lead to deeper relaxation and even the ability to wield a relaxed state more quickly.

- **Try a new teacher.** In yoga, the mindset of *beginner's mind* is encouraged. This means experiencing everything as if for the first time rather than assuming you know the experience already and therefore not bothering to remain present and interested in what is going on in the moment. It is like the old analogy that you can never step foot in the same river twice. The river is always a new river as it is continuously changing moment to moment. Likewise, the practitioner is continuously changing, especially psychologically and therefore every moment is new. It can be very beneficial to learn the basics of yoga from scratch again with a new yoga teacher, if that teacher is of high quality.

- **Use positive reinforcement.** Philosophically speaking, the yoga mindset involves *non-striving*, but at the same time we are doing yoga for specific reasons: Better health etc. So, it is good to remind oneself of why it is worthwhile to practice. Positive goals can be more empowering than negative goals especially in this context. If you practice yoga to *run away* from anxiety you will be practicing a fearful mindset that will potentially become part of your personal identity. So rather than practicing yoga to *run away* from anxiety, practice to *walk towards* serenity and radiance.

- **Don't cage yourself up.** Don't cage yourself up by *trying too hard* to avoid hedonistic pleasures like junk food or smoking. Such interests will normally fall away of their own accord if yoga is practiced regularly for the long term. It is important to watch out for these puritanical traps that can lead to troubles further down the road. Remember, *when you strive you don't become the goal so much as you become the inner-verb that was being practiced along the way to it*. So, if you aim for good health by strictly watching over your own shoulder like a headmaster, that strict character may loom large in your life. Then you may resent yourself further down the track and dive deeper into hedonistic pleasures than ever before.

- **Let go of perfectionism.** The fear of doing things badly will easily stop you from ever doing them well. If you can't do a perfectly tranquil and well-executed yoga session just mess it up however you need to. It's better than getting through the day on sugar instead. And remember, when approaching yoga there is often that basic human aversion to *the unbearable lightness of being*. Put on some loud music if need be and just go through the motions. After twenty minutes or so, you might be in a state that you are ready to turn the music off and sink into the tranquility a little more.

- **High GI foods and stimulants will get in the way.** If you have a lot of refined sugar before a workout it will create more turbulence to fight against as the spike in blood sugar excites the nervous system. This really weakens the effect of yoga. I think of cane sugar as *the yogi's kryptonite.*

- **Sidestep decision fatigue.** Decision fatigue is a real thing and it is crippling people these days more than ever as we have more and more things to say yes or no to. There is so much variety of food, consumer items, social media messages all begging for our attention. To avoid having to make the decision whether to do yoga or not, make a plan that is suited to your lifestyle and stick to it. Don't make the decision on a daily basis, make it on a seasonal basis and stick to it by recalling why it is in your best interests to do so.

- **Make it your own.** If you have a strong distaste for authority you'll probably find it impossible to stick to somebody else's method and routine for the long term. For a person who likes to do things their own way, sticking to a standard routine can create a feeling of being caged up. So, once you've learnt what you want from one teacher, combine it with something else from another art form, or another teacher, or your own intuitive sense of movement and make the workout your own. It will be far more enjoyable this way.

Awareness Trumps Knowledge

"A wealth of information creates a poverty of attention." Herbert Simon, cognitive psychologist

About a decade ago I was studying biomechanics, learning from a professor who was one of the leading researchers in the world when it came to understanding the biomechanics of the spine. Ten years later I saw him walking down the street looking like a walking advertisement for the letter C. Yep, the man with probably the most knowledge of the spine of anybody on the planet had just about the worst spine degeneration I've ever seen. Granted, there may have been genetic factors involved, but I dare say the office working life would have had a lot to do with why he crumpled down so quickly and severely. Knowledge doesn't fix everything.

And very often, when it comes to matters of physical health, awareness trumps knowledge.[xli]

Just as all the information in the world wasn't enough to change the professor's lifestyle, so too, all the nutrition information in the world is not enough to change most people's eating behaviors for the long term and nor will the delivery of an abundance of information get them to exercise effectively.

The intellect doesn't engulf the entire being. It's just a small part of it. You can think to yourself all day—I shouldn't crave that food which is slowly killing me, I shouldn't worry about trivial matters creating unnecessary stress—but the science shows this approach very rarely works.

Why is this so from a neurological perspective? Because the intellectual approach—thinking, using logic, information gathering—relies on a section of the brain called the cortex, and the cortex doesn't have the ability to reduce the stress response for two reasons.xlii First, the cortex doesn't have many direct connections to the amygdala. Second, it is the amygdala that initiates the stress response. Therefore, the effective ways of reducing the stress response and healing anxiety are those that rally with the amygdala. Breathing exercises, meditation and yoga have been found to be effective in such a way.xliii xliv

Breakfast Conspiracies and the Reality of Nutritional Science

Growing up in Australia we were always encouraged to eat cereal for breakfast as if it were the ultimate healthy breakfast. These messages came not just from cereal and milk advertisements but also from the school curriculum which taught the food pyramid with cereals at its base. But does the same thing happen in Japan? Of course not. Japanese people traditionally eat Japanese foods for breakfast, not milk and wheat-based cereal, and yet they are some of the healthiest people on the planet.

Looking into the history of this matter, it turns out that the common acceptance of breakfast cereals into the Western diet originated amongst Seventh Day Adventists. John Harvey Kellogg, one of the founders of 'Adventist health work' developed the concept of breakfast cereals as a health food and that work eventually led to the founding of Kellogg's cereal company by his brother William. Here in Australia, the other dominant cereal brand, Sanitarium Health and Well-Being Company, is also a church owned business. The Adventists believed strongly that cereals really were the ultimate thing to be eating at breakfast time (and for some people it may be true that cereals are the best option) but I do think it's worth taking into account that our education around the first meal of the day has potentially become heavily loaded with economic motives. When one has an incentive to believe something, it can be very easy to believe it. It is not only that the cereal companies are invested in the promotion of cereal but also that the national economies of Australia and North America are heavily invested in wheat production. Once a person develops an incentive for believing something to be true, it can be very hard for them to see alternative perceptions.

In contemplation of the involvement of economic forces in media, advertising and funding of research, other nutrition trivia that might be particularly worth questioning includes, but is not limited to, that surrounding:

- Coffee
- Dairy
- Alcohol
- Meat
- Oils
- Supplements

Many people assume that if something is "supported by science" then it is clearly true. The reality is that only about 17% of scientific research that is published is actually good quality science. The rest is either intentionally misleading for the sake of profiting the funding body, or it is simply poorly conducted methodically.

While there has been plenty of good quality and useful research carried out in the field of nutritional science, nutritional science, in general, is one of the most unreliable fields for two reasons. The first is that the research is often funded by people who are hoping for a particular outcome to be reported. The second is that there are so many variables involved with studying the health effects of diet that it is often very difficult to produce a conclusive scientific result without exaggerating the certainty of the outcome. Nutritional science suffers from a condition known amongst scientists as "physics envy". The term derives from the fact that physics tends to produce a much clearer and more usable outcome than other areas of science tend to do.

As one example of how our knowledge of nutrition is affected by economic factors, consider the dairy industry. Here in Australia we are bombarded with commercials telling us we need milk for its calcium delivery. As a result, many Australians believe that without dairy consumption it is difficult to obtain an adequate intake of calcium. In reality, calcium is found quite abundantly in other foods, especially in some fruits and nuts. Dried figs for example, contain more calcium per weight than cow's milk does. The calcium is easier to metabolize when coming from fruit too.

Some other facts worth considering regarding food and the economy:

- A large fraction of Australia's agricultural industry is devoted to alcohol production; hence it is practically forbidden to criticize beer in this country.

- Regarding oils, many vegetable oils are touted as being superbly healthy and full of nutrition when in reality many are carcinogenic and barely fit for human consumption. It is not that they are lying about the presence of nutritional vitamins and minerals, but that the presence of those factors alone should not verify them as "healthy". House bricks might be high in vitamins and minerals too, but that doesn't mean they're healthy to eat.

- Another big sell is protein. Many supplement products are sold as being high in essential protein. The reality is that your body can only metabolize quite a small amount of protein at each meal (about 25g **maximum**)xlv and it's not so difficult to get the RDI from natural whole foods.

So, while nutritional science can be important when it is carried out with integrity and when the situation calls for it, it isn't *always* the best method of approach. Rather than focusing excessively on *knowledge* of nutrition as a way of coming to a healthy diet, it may be better to keep some basic principles in mind. **Seek medical advice before taking on unusual diets** but as a starting point, some key principles to keep in mind regarding diet are:

1. **That glucocorticoids, the stress hormones mentioned earlier, affect your cravings** and reducing their presence in the body can lead to a healthier appetite.
2. **That gut bacteria affect your brain and your cravings as well as your tendency to gain weight** and eating raw, fibrous whole foods is a good way to foster healthy gut bacteria.[xlvi xlvii xlviii]
3. **That natural whole foods still seem to be the best option** despite that it would be very difficult to sell a trendy book about how to fix your health with this obvious diet.

"Normally, germ-free rodents can eat as much as they like without putting on weight, but this enviable ability disappeared once their guts were colonized. They didn't start eating more food, if anything, they ate slightly less—but they converted more of that food into fat and so piled on the pounds." Ed Yong, Author of 'I Contain Multitudes' xlix

Does More Flexibility Equal Better Health?

Does more flexibility equal better health? Not always. Generally speaking, you want to have quite flexible muscles and tendons provided that those muscles have enough strength to compensate for their flexibility, but your *ligaments* are a whole different story.

For those who are not familiar with the difference between tendons and ligaments—basically *ligaments are the connective tissues that join bone to bone while tendons are the connective tissues that join muscle to bone.*

So, in regard to the knee joint, for example, the ligaments act like the hinges on a door joint allowing it to swing effortlessly and in a firmly controlled fashion. Just as you wouldn't want the hinges of a door to be loosely attached and allowing the door to clumsily flop all over the place as it is being opened or shut, you also don't want the ligaments of the knee to be excessively long as that would lead to unnatural function.

What makes a ligament become too lax? To understand this, it is important to know that ligaments exhibit what biomechanists call *time-dependent-strain.*

Time-dependent-strain means that if you tug on the ligament abruptly the ligament is strong and stiff and holds its length, but if you put even a very light load on a ligament over a long time period (e.g. an hour, or overnight) the ligament stretches and lengthens and can potentially stay like that for some time after the load is removed. The consequence is that you have a joint that is operating ineffectively and this may lead to an acute injury while playing sport for example as the joint is not functioning effectively. It can also lead to excess muscle tension as the muscles need to over-work in order to hold the joint firmly through its range of movement in the way that the ligament would be doing if it were at its healthy length and operating like a firm hinge.

How does this situation happen? The trouble usually begins during rest. Strangely enough, it is most often not the accidents themselves that most often lead to joint problems and muscle problems but rather it is *the way we rest*. For example, it may seem as if you damaged your ACL ligament in your knee during sport but in reality, the situation may have been caused by a knee that was operating unnaturally due to lengthening of the ligament that occurred during an unusual sleep position or sitting position. This is not always the case of course, but it contributes to a great deal of injuries and muscle pains that lead people into the physiotherapists clinic.

In Summary

"The making of minds—and of feelings in particular—is grounded on interactions of the nervous system and its organism. Nervous systems make minds not by themselves but in cooperation with the rest of their own organisms. This is a departure from the traditional view of brains as the sole source of minds." Antonio Damasio, neuroscientist [1]

The practice of Yoga is a time-tested and very effective way of recalibrating the body toward health and a lighter, freer way of living. Many of the outcomes of yoga practice are surprising to most people and the function of yoga is not so woo-woo after all. In fact, any good physiologist can see, rationally, how the myriad benefits of yoga would come about. Embedded in the core philosophy of yoga is an intelligent respect for the interaction between body and mind, though, put more accurately they are not truly separate phenomena. It is not body *and* mind, it is body-mind.

Yoga is a practice that developed independently of any religion and can be tailored to the individual and his or her lifestyle. Its potential for recalibrating the nervous system and resetting (habitually determined) stress levels will be of great interest to many.

Some More Thoughts on Health and Yoga

The Truth About Hip Breakage

Generally speaking, it is a myth that people fall and break their hip. In reality, their hip breaks and they fall as a result of that. The hip had been weakened over time either by cyclic loading, osteoporosis or some other factor.

There is some research to suggest that yoga may reverse osteoporotic bone loss and buffer against the occurrence of bone fractures related to osteoporosis if it is being used as a substitute for more heavy-going activities that would have caused more wear.[li][lii][liii]

Also, if taken up early enough in life, the diet-changing effects of yoga practice may help reduce the risk of osteoporosis also, though this is just my own speculation.

How to Bounce Out of Bed

"Stress not only can decrease the amount of sleep but can also decrease the quality of whatever sleep you do manage." Matthew Walker, Sleep Scientist and Author of 'Why We Sleep'

What is it that causes us to feel so worn out when we wake up in the morning after all that rest? The effect is largely due to blood sugar levels. If there are no interfering medical conditions present, there's a lot you can do about developing the ability to keep healthy blood sugar levels over night. Eating plenty of fiber and avoiding refined carbs is a good starting point.

As a quick guide to a good night's sleep that will help to leave you feeling ready to face the day by morning, the following factors may be useful:

- Eat a healthy amount of fiber
- Avoid refined carbs (as these lead to blood sugar spiking and plummeting)
- Eat cinnamon before bed. This helps to keep blood sugar levels steady over-night.liv 2
- Keep a regular sleep pattern (including on weekends)
- Eat a light meal at dinner and leave at least a couple hours between dinner and bed.

2 (see referenced journal article. You may wish to speak to your doctor before making this a habit)

- Avoid drinking alcohol.

- Practice yoga late in the day (this allows for the body to unwind and makes for a much more relaxed sleep)

- Decide how you will feel in the morning as you go to bed. Making the decision to feel strong, relaxed and confident in the morning and making this decision before going to sleep is sometimes very effective.

- Include a variety of inversion and extension asanas in your yoga practice.

- Interval training or heart-rate variability training develops a kind of fitness that makes it easier to switch modes from sleeping and lying down to getting up and at it.

Cautions

While yoga is a very safe activity relative to many other forms of physical exercise, there are still some risks to keep in mind.

In terms of the physical risks involved, one of the most dangerous asanas is the shoulder stand asana. This asana can lead to various problems for the elderly in particular if there are health problems present or if the shoulder stand has been practiced in an unsafe manner for many years, and so the shoulder stand should be practiced with care and proper training. The Iyengar yoga style addresses this issue by the use of props to make asanas safer. If you intend on practicing the shoulder stand frequently for the long term I recommend taking a beginner's course in Iyengar yoga where they will teach you how to keep your neck safe during the shoulder stand by using props such as blankets, a bolster and a strap as well as using proper technique to alleviate the load on the neck.

84

Another factor to keep in mind is that there have been cases of sexual assault reported in yoga (as is the case with almost every activity) and in particular in kundalini yoga. Kundalini yoga is known to invoke sexual arousal and there have been teachers who have taken advantage of this fact. While many teachers holding courses in kundalini yoga have honest motives, it is important to be aware of kundalini's power to ignite sexual arousal. Kundalini may also be unsafe for people with mental disturbances as the practice may exacerbate such disturbances.

Acknowledgements

I'd like to thank the researchers and writers Robert Sapolsky, Ed Yong, Elizabeth Blackburn, Elissa Epel, Catherine M. Pittman, Elizabeth M. Karle, Ben Goldacre, Antonio Damasio, and William J. Broad, for their writings and influence. Your books and courses are very long and comprehensive and provide a great source of knowledge for those wanting to research the relevant fields in more depth.

For any readers who are wanting to further their knowledge of human behavioral biology I particularly recommend the work of Robert Sapolsky whose courses and books are very entertaining and informative. His free lecture series available on iTunes Podcasts is especially insightful. There is not a boring moment.

Contact Details

To join my email list and keep up to date with my writing, please email me at:

counterintuitivethought@gmail.com

Social Media:

@JaxPaxWorx on Instagram

Recommended Reading

- The Artist's State of Mind: A guide to accessing the flow state by mastery of your chosen craft by Jax Pax
- Why Zebras Don't Get Ulcers by Robert Sapolsky
- The Science of Yoga: The risks and the rewards by William J. Broad
- Rewire Your Anxious Brain: How to use the neuroscience of fear to end anxiety, panic and worry by Catherine M. Pittman and Elizabeth M. Karle
- I Contain Multitudes: The microbes within us and a grander view of life by Ed Yong
- The Telomere Effect by Elizabeth Blackburn and Elissa Epel
- This is Your Brain on Parasites by Kathleen McAuliffe

- The Strange Order of Things: Life, feeling and the making of cultures by Antonio Damasio

- Bad Science by Ben Goldacre

- The Trouble with Testosterone by Robert Sapolsky

- Behave by Robert Sapolsky

- Destructive Emotions: A scientific dialogue with the Dalai Lama by Daniel Goleman and The Mind and Life Institute

- The Mind's Own Physician: A scientific dialogue with the Dalai Lama on the healing power of meditation by Jon Kabat-Zinn and Richard Davidson with Zara Houshmand

- A Physiological Handbook for Teachers of Yogasana by Mel Robin

- A Handbook for Yogasana Teachers: The Incorporation of Neuroscience, Physiology, and Anatomy into the Practice by Mel Robin

Previously by Jax Pax

The Artist's State of Mind: A Guide to Accessing the Flow State by Mastery of Your Chosen Craft

Reviews:

"Australian-born author and songwriter Jax Pax has thought deeply about what happens when we stretch ourselves to the limits of our ability and how it pays off in both quality of performance and enjoyment of what we're doing. He shares more practical wisdom than many much longer books.

Whether you're an artist or a craftsperson, or you want to approach whatever you do with that kind of attention and care, read *The Artist's State of Mind: A Guide to Accessing the Flow State Through Mastery of Your Chosen Craft* slowly and reflectively. Its relaxed prose will speak to you with insights and practices you can apply immediately to achieve mastery of your work and yourself."

Gary Gute
Creativity and Flow Researcher
TheFlowChannel.com

"The Artist's State of Mind by Jax Pax delivers on its title and more. It's short enough to read in one sitting, but

I took a few weeks with it because I admired it as a sound introduction to how artists prepare for their best work, then carry through. Concise. Thoughtful. The author has consolidated lessons from longer works to simplify them for anyone desiring mastery, but this book is particularly friendly to beginners. Pax's observations and insights as a songwriter showcase songwriting as a metaphor for all sorts of creative skills.

Read the table of contents and you'll know if it's for you. I liked it. It reminded me how much attitude affects the work, and that artists can choose a state of mind that calls up creativity."

Marshall Vandruff
Art Teacher and Illustrator
MarshallArt.com and the Proko Channel on YouTube

Reference List

[i] M Hagins, W Moore, A Rundle. 2007. *"Does Practicing Hatha Yoga Satisfy Recommendations for Intensity of Physical Activity Which Improves and Maintains Health and Cardiovascular Fitness?" BMC Complementary Alternative Medicine. Vol 7. 40*

[ii] A L Francis, R C Beemer. 2019. *"How Does Yoga Reduce Stress? Embodied Cognition and Emotion Highlight the Influence of the Musculoskeletal System." Elsevier. Vol 43 pp 170-175*

[iii] S Nair, M Sagar, J Sollers et al. 2015. *"Do Slumped and Upright Postures Affect Stress Responses?" American Psychology Association. Vol 34. 632-641*

[iv] M D Couck, R Caers, L Musch. et al. 2019. *"How Breathing Can Help You Make Better Decisions: Two Studies on the Effects of Breathing Patterns on Heart-Rate Variability and Decision-Making in Business Cases." International Journal of Psychophysiology. Vol 139. pp 1-9*

[v] N Sheiko, V P Feketa. 2019. *'Dynamics of Heart Rate Variability Under the Influence of Course Yoga Breathing Exercises on Healthy Young People'. via PubMed. 72 (4), 613-616*

vi Sapolsky, R., 2004. Why Zebras Don't Get Ulcers: The acclaimed guide to stress, stress-related diseases, and coping. 3rd ed. New York: Henry Holt and Company, LLC.

vii M. Campos MD, 2017, *Heart Rate Variability: A New Way to Track Well-being,* Harvard Health Publishing. https://www.health.harvard.edu/blog/heart-rate-variability-new-way-track-well-2017112212789

viii M E B Russell, A B Scott, I A Boggero, C R Carlson. 2017. *"Inclusion of a Rest Period in Diaphragmatic Breathing Increases High Frequency Heart Rate Variability: Implications for Behavioural Therapy." Psychophysiology. Vol 54. pp 358-365*

ix L Zou, J E Sasaki, G Wei, T Huang, A S Yeung, O B Neto, K W Chen, S S Hui. 2018. *'Effects of Mind-Body Exercises (Tai-Chi/Yoga) on Heart Rate Variability Parameters and Perceived Stress: A Systematic Review with Meta-Analysis of Randomized Controlled Trials.' PubMed.* 10.3390/jcm7110404

x A Tyagi, M Cohen. 2016. *'Yoga and Heart Rate Variability: A Comprehensive Review of the Literature.' International Journal of Yoga accessed via PubMed.* 10.4103/0973-6131.183712

xi V C Goessl, J E Curtis, SG Hofmann. 2017. *'The Effect of Heart Rate Variability Biofeedback*

Training on Stress and Anxiety: A Meta-Analysis'. PubMed. 47. (15), 2578-2586

[xii] C C Streeter, J E Jensen, R M Perlmutter, H J Cabral, H Tian, D B Terhune, D A Ciraulo, P F Renshaw. 2007. *'Yoga Asana Sessions Increase Brain GABA Levels: A Pilot Study.' Journal of Alternative and Complementary Medicine Accessed via PubMed.* 10.1089/acm.2007.6338

[xiii] C C Streeter, P L Gerbarg, R P Brown, T M Scott, G H Nielsen, L Owen, O Sakai, J T Sneider, M B Nyer, M M Silveri. 2020. *'Thalamic Gamma Aminobutyric Acid Level Changes in Major Depressive Disorder After a 12-Week Iyengar and Coherent Breathing Intervention.' Journal of Alternative and Complementary Medicine Accessed via PubMed.* 10.1089/acm.2019.0234

[xiv] Sapolsky R, 2010. Human Behavioural Biology: Aggression II lecture. Accessed via iTunes podcasts.

[xv] C C Streeter, J E Jensen, R M Perlmutter, H J Cabral, H Tian, D B Terhune, D A Ciraulo, P F Renshaw. 2007. *'Yoga Asana Sessions Increase Brain GABA Levels: A Pilot Study.' Journal of Alternative and Complementary Medicine Accessed via PubMed.* 10.1089/acm.2007.6338

[xvi] C C Streeter, T H Whitfield, L Owen, T Rein, S K Karri, A Yakhkind, R Perlmutter, A Prescot, P F Renshaw, D A Ciraulo, J E Jensen. 2010.

'Effects of Yoga Versus Walking on Mood, Anxiety, and Brain GABA Levels: A Randomized Controlled MRS Study.' Journal of Alternative and Complementary Medicine. 10.1089/acm.2010.0007

xvii Sapolsky, R., 2004. Why Zebras Don't Get Ulcers: The acclaimed guide to stress, stress-related diseases, and coping. 3rd ed. New York: Henry Holt and Company, LLC.

xviii S H Park, K S Han. 2017. *Blood Pressure Response to Meditation and Yoga: A Systematic Review and Meta-Analysis.' Journal of Alternative and Complementary Medicine via PubMed.* 10.1089/acm.2016.0234.

xix S Telles, S Verma, S K Sharma, R K Gupta, A Balkrishna. 2017. *'Alternate-Nostril Yoga Breathing Reduced Blood Pressure While Increasing Performance in a Vigilance Test.' Medical Science Monitor Basic Research via PubMed.* 10.12659/msmbr.906502

xx M C Pascoe, D R Thompson, C F Ski. 2017. *'Yoga, Mindfulness-Based Stress Reduction and Stress-Related Physiological Measures: A Meta-Analysis.' Psychoneuroendocrinology via PubMed.* 10.1016/j.psyneuen.2017.08.008.

xxi D L Cohen, L T Bloedon, R L Rothman, J T Farrar, M L Galantino, S Volger, C Mayor, P O Szapary, R R Townsend. 2011. *'Iyengar Yoga Versus Enhanced Usual Care on Blood Pressure in Patients with Prehypertension to Stage 1 Hypertension: A Randomized Controlled Trial.' Evidence Based Complementary Alternative Medicine via PubMed.* 10.1093/ecam/nep130

xxii S Levenstein, M W Smith, G A Kaplan. 2001. *'Psychosocial Predictors of Hypertension in Men and Women.' Arch Internal Medicine via PubMed.* 161(10):1341-6

xxiii Sapolsky, R., 1997. The Trouble with Testosterone: And other essays on the biology of the human predicament. 1st ed. New York: Scribner.

xxiv Sapolsky, R., 2004. Why Zebras Don't Get Ulcers: The acclaimed guide to stress, stress-related diseases, and coping. 3rd ed. New York: Henry Holt and Company, LLC.

xxv Sapolsky, R., 2004. Why Zebras Don't Get Ulcers: The acclaimed guide to stress, stress-related diseases, and coping. 3rd ed. New York: Henry Holt and Company, LLC.

xxvi Sapolsky, R., 1997. The Trouble with Testosterone: And other essays on the biology of the human predicament. 1st ed. New York: Scribner.

xxvii J D Gode, R H Singh, R M Settiwar, et al. 1974. *'Increased Urinary Excretion of Testosterone Following a Course of Yoga in*

Normal Young Volunteers.' Indian Journal of Medical Sciences, vol. 28

xxviii R S Minvaleev, A D Nozdrachev, V V Kiryanova, et al. 2004. *"Postural Influences on the Hormone Level in Healthy Subjects: I. The Cobra Posture and Steroid Hormones," Human Physiology, vol. 30, no. 4 pp. 452–56.*

xxix Sapolsky, R., 2004. Why Zebras Don't Get Ulcers: The acclaimed guide to stress, stress-related diseases, and coping. 3rd ed. New York: Henry Holt and Company, LLC.

xxx Damasio, A., 2018. The Strange Order of Things: Life, Feeling and the Making of Cultures. 1st ed. Toronto: Pantheon Books

xxxi Sapolsky, R., 2004. Why Zebras Don't Get Ulcers: The acclaimed guide to stress, stress-related diseases, and coping. 3rd ed. New York: Henry Holt and Company, LLC.

xxxii Sapolsky, R., 2004. Why Zebras Don't Get Ulcers: The acclaimed guide to stress, stress-related diseases, and coping. 3rd ed. New York: Henry Holt and Company, LLC.

xxxiii Sapolsky, R., 2004. Why Zebras Don't Get Ulcers: The acclaimed guide to stress, stress-related diseases, and coping. 3rd ed. New York: Henry Holt and Company, LLC.

xxxiv Blackburn E, Epel E, 2017. The Telomere Effect: A revolutionary approach to living younger, healthier, longer. 1st ed. London: Orion Spring

xxxv D Ornish, J Lin, J Daubenmier, et al. 2008. *"Increased Telomerase Activity and Comprehensive Lifestyle Changes: A Pilot Study," Lancet Oncology, vol. 9, no. 11 pp. 1048–57.*

xxxvi Q A Conklin, B G King, A P Zanesco, et al. 2018. *"Insight Meditation and Telomere Biology: The Effects of Intensive Retreat and the Moderating Role of Personality." Elsevier, vol. 70, pp. 233-245.*

xxxvii Y Lu, B Rosner, G Chang, L M Fishman. 2016. *"Twelve-Minute Daily Yoga Regimen Reverses Osteoporotic Bone Loss." Lippincott Williams and Wilkins, vol 32. 81-87*

xxxviii Broad W J, 2012. The Science of Yoga: The Risks and the Rewards. 1st ed. New York: Simon and Schuster

xxxix Sapolsky R, 2010. Human Behavioural Biology: Aggression II lecture. Accessed via iTunes podcasts.

xl Sapolsky, R., 2004. Why Zebras Don't Get Ulcers: The acclaimed guide to stress, stress-related diseases, and coping. 3rd ed. New York: Henry Holt and Company, LLC.

xli (Which is why this book is very short by comparison to most nonfiction science books.)

[xlii] Pittman C M, Karle E M, 2015. Rewire Your Anxious Brain: How to Use the Neuroscience of Fear to End Anxiety, Panic and Worry. 1st ed. Oakland: New Harbinger Publications, Inc.

[xliii] R Jerath, V A Barnes, D Dillard-Wright, et al. 2012. *"Dynamic Change of Awareness During Meditation Techniques: Neural and Physiological Correlates." Frontiers in Human Neuroscience, vol. 6: 131*

[xliv] Pittman C M, Karle E M, 2015. Rewire Your Anxious Brain: How to Use the Neuroscience of Fear to End Anxiety, Panic and Worry. 1st ed. Oakland: New Harbinger Publications, Inc.

[xlv] B J Schoenfeld, A A Aragon, 2018. *"How Much Protein Can the Body Use in a Single Meal for Muscle-Building? Implications for Daily Protein Distribution." Journal of the International Society of Sports Nutrition, vol 15: 10*

[xlvi] Long E, 2016. I contain Multitudes: The Microbes Within Us and a Grander View of Life. 1st ed. London: Bodley Head

[xlvii] S O Fettisov. 2017. *"Role of the Gut Microbiota in Host Appetite Control: Bacterial Growth to Animal Feeding Behavior." Nature Reviews Endocrinology, vol 13 (1), pp 11-25*

[xlviii] M Wouw, H Schellekens, et al. 2017. *"Microbiota-Gut-Brain Axis: Modulator of Host*

Metabolism and Appetite." Journal of Nutrition, vol 147 (5), pp 727-745

xlix Long E, 2016. I contain Multitudes: The Microbes Within Us and a Grander View of Life. 1st ed. London: Bodley Head

l Damasio, A., 2018. The Strange Order of Things: Life, Feeling and the Making of Cultures. 1st ed. Toronto: Pantheon Books

li E N Smith, A Boser. 2013. *"Yoga, Vertebral Fractures, and Osteoporosis: Research and Recommendations." International Journal of Yoga Therapy. vol 23 1 17-23*

lii Z S Motorwala, S Kolke, P Y Panchal, et al. 2016. *"Effects of Yogasanas on Osteoporosis in Postmenopausal Women." International Journal of Yoga. vol 9 (1), 44-48*

liii Y Lu, B Rosner, G Chang, L M Fishman. 2016. *"Twelve-Minute Daily Yoga Regimen Reverses Osteoporotic Bone Loss." Lippincott Williams and Wilkins, vol 32. 81-87*

liv T Lu, H Sheng, J Wu, et al. 2012. *"Cinnamon Extract Improves Fasting Blood Glucose and Glycosylated Hemoglobin Level in Chinese Patients with Type-2 Diabetes." Nutritional Research, vol 32 (6), pp 408-412.*